Keto Vegetarian Cookbook

Ketogenic Recipes for Vegetarians for Weight Loss and a Healthy Lifestyle

Ricardo Abagnale

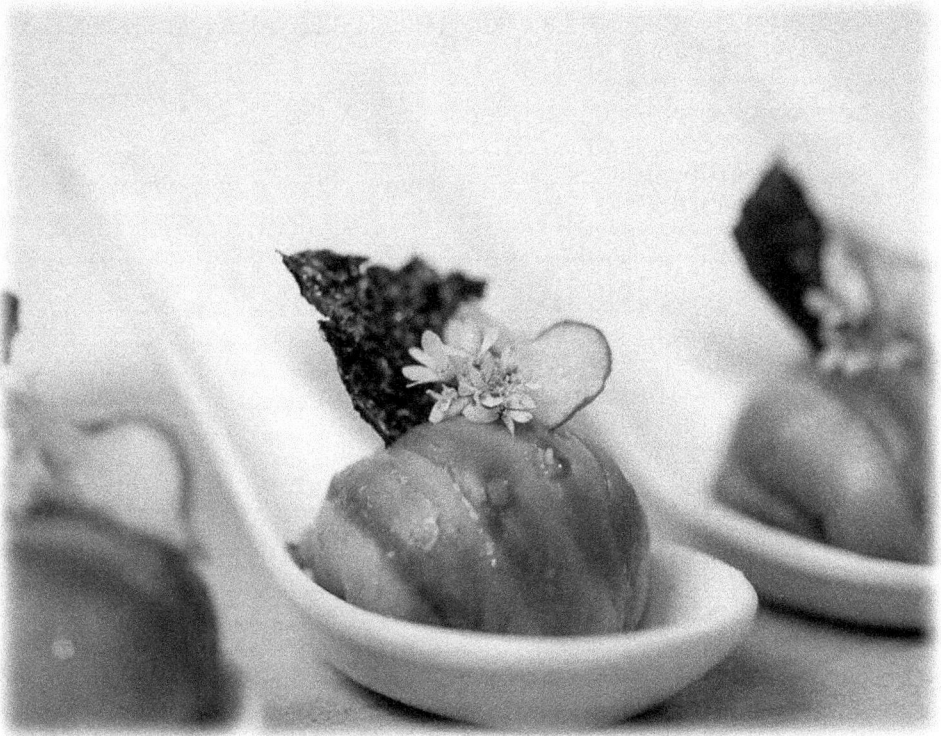

Table of Contents

INTRODUCTION

The Ketogenic diet is truly life changing. The diet improves your overall health and helps you lose the extra weight in a matter of days. The diet will show its multiple benefits even from the beginning and it will become your new lifestyle really soon.

As soon as you embrace the Ketogenic diet, you will start to live a completely new life.

On the other hand, the vegetarian diet is such a healthy dietary option you can choose when trying to live healthy and also lose some weight.

The collection we bring to you today is actually a combination between the Ketogenic and vegetarian diets. You get to discover some amazing Ketogenic vegetarian dishes you can prepare in the comfort of your own home. All the dishes you found here follow both the Ketogenic and the vegetarian rules, they all taste delicious and rich and they are all easy to make.

We can assure you that such a combo is hard to find. So, start a keto diet with a vegetarian "touch" today. It will be both useful and fun!

So, what are you still waiting for? Get started with the Ketogenic diet and learn how to prepare the best and most flavored Ketogenic vegetarian dishes. Enjoy them all!

Mint Watermelon Bowl

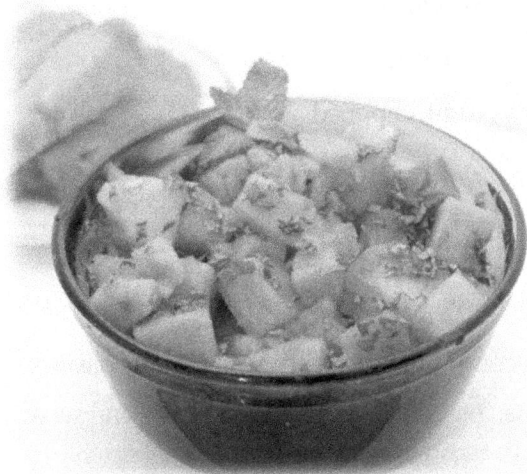

Preparation time: 5 minutes

Cooking time: 0 minutes

Servings: 2

Nutritional Values (Per Serving):

- Calories 90
- Fat 3
- Fiber 1
- Carbs 7
- Protein 2

Ingredients:

- 2 cups watermelon, peeled and cubed
- 6 kalamata olives, pitted and sliced
- 1 teaspoon avocado oil
- ½ tablespoon balsamic vinegar
- 1 tablespoon mint, chopped

Directions:

1. In a bowl, combine the watermelon with the olives and the other ingredients, toss, divide into smaller bowls and serve.

Roasted Peppers Muffins

Preparation time: 10 minutes

Cooking time: 15 minutes

Servings: 6

Nutritional Values (Per Serving):

- Calories 209
- Fat 16.7
- Fiber 1.8
- Carbs 6.8
- Protein 9.3

Ingredients:

- 2 tablespoons flaxseed mixed with 3 tablespoons water
- 1/3 cup spinach, chopped
- ½ cup coconut cream
- ¼ cup cashew cheese, grated
- ½ cup roasted red peppers, chopped
- A pinch of salt and black pepper
- 2 tablespoons oregano, chopped
- 1 teaspoon chili powder
- Cooking spray

Directions:

1. In a bowl, combine the spinach with the flaxseed mix, the cream and the other ingredients except the cooking spray, and whisk well.

2. Grease a muffin pan with the cooking spray, divide the peppers mix, bake at 400 degrees F for 15 minutes and serve for breakfast.

Tomato and Avocado Pizza

Preparation time: 20 minutes

Cooking time: 20 minutes

Servings: 2

Nutritional Values (Per Serving):

- Calories 416
- Fat 24.5
- Fiber 9.6
- Carbs 36.6
- Protein 15.4

Ingredients:

- 2 cups almond flour
- A pinch of salt and black pepper
- 1 and ½ cups water
- 2 tablespoons avocado oil
- 1 teaspoon chili powder
- 1 tomato, sliced
- 1 avocado, peeled, pitted and sliced
- ¼ cup tomato passata
- 2 tablespoons chives, chopped

Directions:

1. In a bowl, mix the flour with salt, pepper, water, the oil and chili powder, stir well until you obtain a dough, knead a bit, put in a bowl, cover and leave aside for 20 minutes.
2. Transfer the dough to a working surface, shape a circle, transfer it to a baking sheet lined with parchment paper and bake at 400 degrees F for 10 minutes.
3. Spread the tomato passata over the pizza crust, also add the rest of the ingredients and bake at 400 degrees F for 10 minutes more.
4. Cut and serve for breakfast.

Creamy Brussels Sprouts Bowls

Preparation time: 10 minutes

Cooking time: 30 minutes

Servings: 4

Nutritional Values (Per Serving):

- Calories 219
- Fat 18.3
- Fiber 5.7
- Carbs 14.1
- Protein 5.4

Ingredients:

- 1 tablespoon olive oil
- 2 pound Brussels sprouts, trimmed and halved
- 1 cup coconut cream
- ½ teaspoon chili powder

- ½ teaspoon garam masala
- ½ teaspoon garlic powder
- A pinch of salt and black pepper
- 1 tablespoon lime juice

Directions:

1. In a roasting pan, combine the sprouts with the cream, chili powder and the other ingredients, toss, introduce in the oven at 380 degrees F and bake for 30 minutes.
2. Divide into bowls and serve for lunch.

Green Beans and Radishes Bake

Preparation time: 10 minutes

Cooking time: 25 minutes

Servings: 4

Nutritional Values (Per Serving):

- Calories 130
- Fat 1
- Fiber 0.4
- Carbs 1
- Protein 0.1

Ingredients:

- 2 tablespoons olive oil
- 1 pound green beans, trimmed
- halved 2 cups radishes, sliced
- 1 cup coconut cream
- 1 teaspoon sweet paprika
- 1 cup cashew cheese, shredded
- Salt and black pepper to the taste

- 1 tablespoon chives, chopped

Directions:

1. In a roasting pan, combine the green beans with the radishes and the other ingredients except the cheese and toss.
2. Sprinkle the cheese on top, introduce in the oven at 375 degrees F and bake for 25 minutes.
3. Divide the mix between plates and serve.

Avocado and Radish Bowls

Preparation time: 10 minutes

Cooking time: 0 minutes

Servings: 4

Nutritional Values (Per Serving):

- Calories 340
- Fat 23
- Fiber 3
- Carbs 6
- Protein 5

Ingredients:

- 2 cups radishes, halved
- 2 avocados, peeled, pitted and roughly cubed
- 2 tablespoons coconut cream
- 2 tablespoons balsamic vinegar
- 1 tablespoon green onion, chopped
- 1 teaspoon chili powder

- 1 cup baby spinach
- Salt and black pepper to the taste

Directions:

1. In a bowl, combine the radishes with the avocados and the other ingredients, toss, divide into smaller bowls and serve for lunch.

Celery and Radish Soup

Preparation time: 10 minutes

Cooking time: 20 minutes

Servings: 4

Nutritional Values (Per Serving):

- Calories 120
- Fat 2
- Fiber 1
- Carbs 3
- Protein 10

Ingredients:

- ½ pound radishes, cut into quarters
- 2 celery stalks, chopped
- 2 tablespoons olive oil
- 4 scallions, chopped
- 1 teaspoon fennel seeds, crushed
- 1 teaspoon coriander, dried
- 6 cups vegetable stock

- Salt and black pepper to the taste
- 6 garlic cloves, minced
- 1 tablespoon chives, chopped

Directions:

1. Heat up a pot with the oil over medium heat, add the celery, scallions and the garlic and sauté for 5 minutes.
2. Add the radishes and the other ingredients, bring to a boil, cover and simmer for 15 minutes.
3. Divide into soup bowls and serve.

Lime Avocado and Cucumber Soup

Preparation time: 5 minutes

Cooking time: 0 minutes

Servings: 4

Nutritional Values (Per Serving):

- Calories 100
- Fat 10
- Fiber 2
- Carbs 5
- Protein 8

Ingredients:

- 2 avocados, pitted, peeled and roughly cubed
- 2 cucumbers, sliced
- 4 cups vegetable stock
- Salt and black pepper to the taste
- ¼ teaspoon lemon zest, grated

- 1 tablespoon white vinegar
- 1 cup scallions, chopped
- 1 tablespoon olive oil
- ¼ cup cilantro, chopped

Directions:

1. In a blender, combine the avocados with the cucumbers and the other ingredients, pulse well, divide into bowls and serve for lunch.

Avocado and Kale Soup

Preparation time: 5 minutes

Cooking time: 7 minutes

Servings: 4

Nutritional Values (Per Serving):

- Calories 234
- Fat 12
- Fiber 4
- Carbs 7
- Protein 12

Ingredients:

- 4 cups kale, torn
- 1 teaspoon turmeric powder
- 1 avocado, pitted, peeled and sliced 4 cups vegetable stock
- Juice of 1 lime
- 2 garlic cloves, minced
- 1 tablespoon chives, chopped Salt and black pepper to the taste

Directions:

1. In a pot, combine the kale with the avocado and the other ingredients, bring to a simmer, cook over medium heat for 7 minutes, blend using an immersion blender, divide into bowls and serve.

Spinach and Cucumber Salad

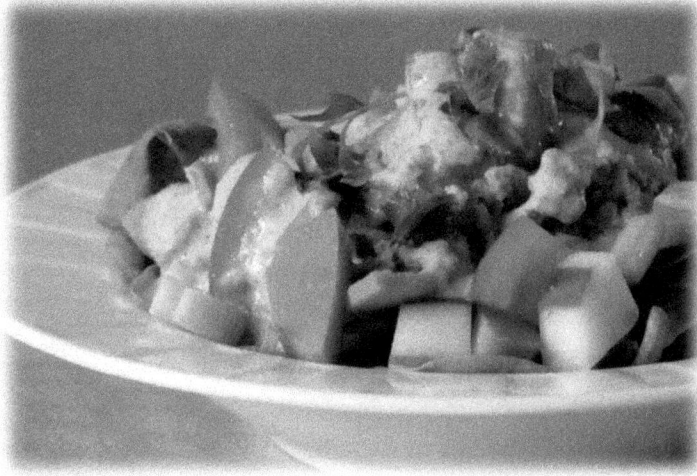

Preparation time: 5 minutes

Cooking time: 0 minutes

Servings: 4

Nutritional Values (Per Serving):

- Calories 140
- Fat 4
- Fiber 2
- Carbs 4
- Protein 5

Ingredients:

- 1 pound cucumber, sliced 2 cups baby spinach
- 1 tablespoon chili powder 2 tablespoons olive oil
- ¼ cup cilantro, chopped
- 2 tablespoons lemon juice
- Salt and black pepper to the taste

Directions:

1. In a large salad bowl, combine the cucumber with the spinach and the other ingredients, toss and serve for lunch.

Curry Spinach Soup

Preparation time: 10 minutes

Cooking time: 0 minutes

Servings: 4

Nutritional Values (Per Serving):

- Calories 240
- Fat 4
- Fiber 2
- Carbs 6
- Protein 2

Ingredients:

- 1 cup almond milk
- 1 tablespoon green curry paste
- 1 pound spinach leaves
- 1 tablespoon cilantro, chopped
- Salt and black pepper to the taste
- 4 cups veggie stock

Directions:

1. In your blender, combine the almond milk with the curry paste and the other ingredients, pulse well, divide into bowls and serve for lunch.

Basil Zucchinis and Eggplants

Preparation time: 10 minutes

Cooking time: 20 minutes

Servings: 4

Nutritional Values (Per Serving):

- Calories 97
- Fat 4
- Fiber 2
- Carbs 6
- Protein 2

Ingredients:

- 1 tablespoon olive oil
- 2 zucchinis, sliced
- 1 eggplant, roughly cubed
- 2 scallions, chopped

- 1 tablespoon sweet paprika
- Juice of 1 lime
- 1 teaspoon fennel seeds, crushed
- Salt and black pepper to the taste
- 1 tablespoon basil, chopped

Directions:

1. Heat up a pan with the oil over medium heat, add the scallions and fennel seeds and sauté for 5 minutes.
2. Add zucchinis, eggplant and the other ingredients, toss, cook over medium heat for 15 minutes more, divide between plates and serve as a side dish.

Chard and Peppers Mix

Preparation time: 10 minutes

Cooking time: 20 minutes

Servings: 4

Nutritional Values (Per Serving):

- Calories 119
- Fat 7
- Fiber 3
- Carbs 7
- Protein 2

Ingredients:

- 2 tablespoons avocado oil
- 2 spring onions, chopped
- 2 tablespoons tomato passata
- 2 tablespoons capers, drained
- 2 green bell peppers, cut into strips
- 1 teaspoon turmeric powder
- A pinch of cayenne pepper

- Juice of 1 lime
- Salt and black pepper to the taste
- 1 bunch red chard, torn

Directions:

1. Heat up a pan with the oil over medium heat, add the spring onions, capers, turmeric and cayenne and sauté for 5 minutes.
2. Add the peppers, chard and the other ingredients, toss, cook over medium heat for 15 minutes more, divide between plates and serve.

Balsamic Kale

Preparation time: 10 minutes

Cooking time: 20 minutes

Servings: 4

Nutritional Values (Per Serving):

- Calories 170
- Fat 11
- Fiber 3
- Carbs 7
- Protein 7

Ingredients:

- 1 tablespoon balsamic vinegar
- 2 tablespoons walnuts, chopped
- 1 pound kale, torn
- 1 tablespoon olive oil
- 1 teaspoon cumin, ground
- 1 teaspoon chili powder

- 3 garlic cloves, minced
- 2 tablespoons cilantro, chopped

Directions:

1. Heat up a pan with the oil over medium heat, add the garlic and the walnuts and cook for 2 minutes.
2. Add the kale, vinegar and the other ingredients, toss, cook over medium heat for 18 minutes more, divide between plates and serve as a side.

Mustard Cabbage Salad

Preparation time: 10 minutes

Cooking time: 0 minutes

Servings: 4

Nutritional Values (Per Serving):

- Calories 150
- Fat 3
- Fiber 2
- Carbs 2
- Protein 7

Ingredients:

- 1 green cabbage head, shredded
- 1 red cabbage head, shredded
- 2 tablespoons avocado oil
- 2 tablespoons mustard
- 1 tablespoon balsamic vinegar
- 1 teaspoon hot paprika

- Salt and black pepper to the taste
- 1 tablespoon dill, chopped

Directions:

1. In a bowl, mix the cabbage with the oil, mustard and the other ingredients, toss, divide between plates and serve as a side salad.

Cabbage and Green Beans

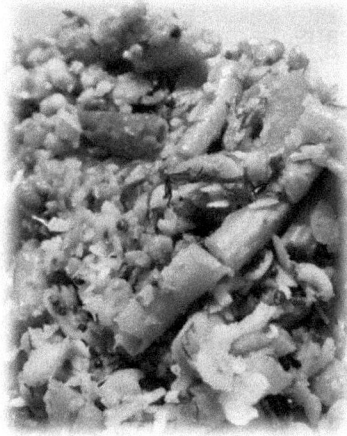

Preparation time: 10 minutes

Cooking time: 15 minutes

Servings: 4

Nutritional Values (Per Serving):

- Calories 200
- Fat 4
- Fiber 2
- Carbs 3
- Protein 7

Ingredients:

- 1 green cabbage head, shredded
- 2 cups green beans, trimmed and halved
- 2 tablespoons olive oil
- 1 teaspoon sweet paprika
- 1 teaspoon cumin, ground
- Salt and black pepper to the taste
- 1 tablespoon chives, chopped

Directions:

1. Heat up a pan with the oil over medium heat, add the cabbage and the paprika and sauté for 2 minutes.
2. Add the green beans and the other ingredients, toss, cook over medium heat fro 13 minutes more, divide between plates and serve.

Green Beans, Avocado and Scallions

Preparation time: 10 minutes

Cooking time: 20 minutes

Servings: 4

Nutritional Values (Per Serving):

- Calories 200
- Fat 5
- Fiber 2,3
- Carbs 1
- Protein 3

Ingredients:

- 1 pound green beans, trimmed and halved
- 1 avocado, peeled, pitted and sliced
- 4 scallions, chopped
- 2 tablespoons olive oil
- 1 tablespoon lime juice

- Salt and black pepper to the taste
- A handful cilantro, chopped

Directions:

1. Heat up a pan with the oil over medium heat, add the scallions and sauté for 2 minutes.
2. Add the green beans, lime juice and the other ingredients, toss, cook over medium heat for 18 minutes, divide between plates and serve.

Grilled Portobello with Mashed Potatoes and Green Beans

Preparation time: 20 minutes

Cooking time: 40 minutes

Servings: 4

Nutritional Values (Per Serving):

- Calories: 263
- Total fat: 7g
- Carbs: 43g
- Fiber: 7g
- Protein: 10g

Ingredients:

For the grilled portobellos

- 4 large portobello mushrooms
- 1 teaspoon olive oil
- Pinch sea salt

For the mashed potatoes

- 6 large potatoes, scrubbed or peeled, and chopped
- 3 to 4 garlic cloves, minced
- ½ teaspoon olive oil
- ½ cup non-dairy milk
- 2 tablespoons coconut oil (optional
- 2 tablespoons nutritional yeast (optional Pinch sea salt)

For the green beans

- 2 cups green beans, cut into 1-inch pieces
- 2 to 3 teaspoons coconut oil
- Pinch sea salt
- 1 to 2 tablespoons nutritional yeast (optional)

Directions:

For the Grilled Portobellos

1. Preheat the grill to medium, or the oven to 350°F.
2. Take the stems out of the mushrooms.
3. Wipe the caps clean with a damp paper towel, then dry them. Spray the caps with a bit of olive oil, or put some oil in your hand and rub it over the mushrooms. Rub the oil onto the top and bottom of each mushroom, then sprinkle them with a bit of salt on top and bottom.
4. Put them bottom side facing up on a baking sheet in the oven, or straight on the grill. They'll take about 30 minutes in the

oven, or 20 minutes on the grill. Wait until they're soft and wrinkling around the edges. If you keep them bottom up, all the delicious mushroom juice will pool in the cap. Then at the very end, you can flip them over to drain the juice. If you like it, you can drizzle it over the mashed potatoes.

For the Mashed Potatoes

5. Boil the chopped potatoes in lightly salted water for about 20 minutes, until soft. While they're cooking, sauté the garlic in the olive oil, or bake them whole in a 350°F oven for 10 minutes, then squeeze out the flesh. Drain the potatoes, reserving about ½ cup water to mash them. In a large bowl, mash the potatoes with a little bit of the reserved water, the cooked garlic, milk, coconut oil (if using), nutritional yeast (if using), and salt to taste. Add more water, a little at a time, if needed, to get the texture you want. If you use an immersion blender or beater to purée them, you'll have some extra-creamy potatoes.

For the Green Bean

6. Heat a medium pot with a small amount of water to boil, then steam the green beans by either putting them directly in the pot or in a steaming basket.

7. Once they're slightly soft and vibrantly green, 7 to 8 minutes, take them off the heat and toss them with the oil, salt, and nutritional yeast (if using).

Tahini Broccoli Slaw

Preparation time: 15 minutes

Cooking time: 0 minutes

Servings: 4 to 6

Ingredients:

- ¼ cup tahini (sesame paste)
- 2 tablespoons white miso
- 1 tablespoon rice vinegar
- 1 tablespoon toasted sesame oil
- 2 teaspoons soy sauce
- 1 (12-ouncebag broccoli slaw)
- 2 green onions, minced
- ¼ cup toasted sesame seeds

Directions:

1. In a large bowl, whisk together the tahini, miso, vinegar, oil, and soy sauce. Add the broccoli slaw, green onions, and sesame seeds and toss to coat.
2. Set aside for 20 minutes before serving.

Steamed Cauliflower

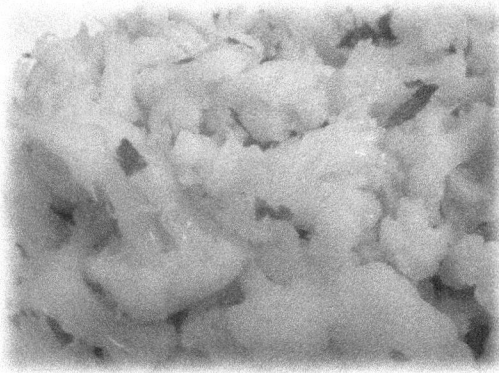

Preparation time: 5 minutes

Cooking time: 10 minutes

Servings: 6

Nutritional Values (Per Serving):

- Calories: 35
- Fat: 0g
- Protein: 3g
- Carbohydrates: 7g
- Fiber: 4g
- Sugar: 4g
- Sodium: 236mg

Ingredients:

- 1 large head cauliflower
- 1 cup water
- ½ teaspoon salt
- 1 teaspoon red pepper flakes (optional)

Directions:

1. Remove any leaves from the cauliflower, and cut it into florets.
2. In a large saucepan, bring the water to a boil. Place a steamer basket over the water, and add the florets and salt. Cover and steam for 5 to 7 minutes, until tender. In a large bowl, toss the cauliflower with the red pepper flakes (if using). Transfer the florets to a large airtight container or 6 single-serving containers. Let cool before sealing the lids.

Roasted Cauliflower Tacos

Preparation time: 10 minutes

Cooking time: 30 minutes

Servings: 8 tacos

Nutrition (1 taco):

- Calories: 198
- Total fat: 6g
- Carbs: 32g
- Fiber: 6g
- Protein: 7g

Ingredients:

For the roasted cauliflower

- 1 head cauliflower, cut into bite-size pieces
- 1 tablespoon olive oil (optional
- 2 tablespoons whole-wheat flour
- 2 tablespoons nutritional yeast

For the tacos

- 1 to 2 teaspoons smoked paprika
- ½ to 1 teaspoon chili powder Pinch sea salt
- 2 cups shredded lettuce
- 2 cups cherry tomatoes, quartered
- 2 carrots, scrubbed or peeled, and grated
- ½ cup Fresh Mango Salsa
- ½ cup Guacamole
- 8 small whole-grain or corn tortillas 1 lime, cut into 8 wedges

Directions:

For the Roasted Cauliflower

1. Preheat the oven to 350°F. Lightly grease a large rectangular baking sheet with olive oil, or line it with parchment paper. In a large bowl, toss the cauliflower pieces with oil (if using), or just rinse them so they're wet. The idea is to get the seasonings to stick. In a smaller bowl, mix together the flour, nutritional yeast, paprika, chili powder, and salt.
2. Add the seasonings to the cauliflower, and mix it around with your hands to thoroughly coat. Spread the cauliflower on the baking sheet, and roast for 20 to 30 minutes, or until softened.

For the Tacos.

3. Prep the veggies, salsa, and guacamole while the cauliflower is roasting. Once the cauliflower is cooked, heat the tortillas for just a few minutes in the oven or in a small skillet. Set everything out on the table, and assemble your tacos as you go. Give a squeeze of fresh lime just before eating.

Cajun Sweet Potatoes

Preparation time: 5 minutes

Cooking time: 30 minutes

Servings: 4

Nutritional Values (Per Serving):

- Calories: 219
- Fat: 3g
- Protein: 4g
- Carbohydrates: 46g
- Fiber: 7g
- Sugar: 9g
- Sodium: 125mg

Ingredients:

- 2 pounds sweet potatoes
- 2 teaspoons extra-virgin olive oil
- ½ teaspoon ground cayenne pepper
- ½ teaspoon smoked paprika
- ½ teaspoon dried oregano

- ½ teaspoon dried thyme
- ½ teaspoon garlic powder
- ½ teaspoon salt (optional

Directions:

1. Preheat the oven to 400°F. Line a baking sheet with parchment paper.
2. Wash the potatoes, pat dry, and cut into ¾-inch cubes. Transfer to a large bowl, and pour the olive oil over the potatoes.
3. In a small bowl, combine the cayenne, paprika, oregano, thyme, and garlic powder. Sprinkle the spices over the potatoes and combine until the potatoes are well coated. Spread the potatoes on the prepared baking sheet in a single layer. Season with the salt (if using). Roast for 30 minutes, stirring the potatoes after 15 minutes.
4. Divide the potatoes evenly among 4 single-serving containers. Let cool completely before sealing.

Creamy Mint-Lime Spaghetti Squash

Preparation time: 10 minutes

Cooking time: 30 minutes

Servings: 3

Nutritional Values (Per Serving):

- Calories: 199
- Total fat: 10g
- Carbs: 27g
- Fiber: 5g
- Protein: 7g

Ingredients:

For the dressing

- 3 tablespoons tahini
- Zest and juice of 1 small lime
- 2 tablespoons fresh mint, minced

- 1 small garlic clove, pressed
- 1 tablespoon nutritional yeast
- Pinch sea salt

For the spaghetti squash

- 1 spaghetti squash
- Pinch sea salt
- 1 cup cherry tomatoes, chopped
- 1 cup chopped bell pepper, any color
- Freshly ground black pepper

Directions:

For the Dressing

1. Make the dressing by whisking together the tahini and lime juice until thick, stirring in water if you need it, until smooth, then add the rest of the Ingredients. Or you can purée all the Ingredients in a blender.

For the Spaghetti Squash.

2. Put a large pot of water on high and bring to a boil. Cut the squash in half and scoop out the seeds. Put the squash halves in the pot with the salt, and boil for about 30 minutes. Carefully remove the squash from the pot and let it cool until you can safely handle it. Set half the squash aside for another

meal. Scoop out the squash from the skin, which stays hard like a shell, and break the strands apart. The flesh absorbs water while boiling, so set the "noodles" in a strainer for 10 minutes, tossing occasionally to drain. Transfer the cooked spaghetti squash to a large bowl and toss with the mint-lime dressing. Then top with the cherry tomatoes and bell pepper. Add an extra sprinkle of nutritional yeast and black pepper, if you wish.

Black Bean Soup

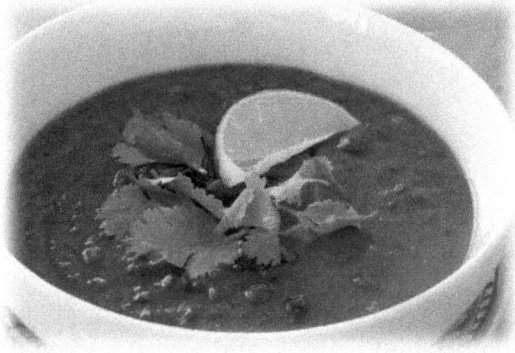

Preparation time: 10 minutes

Cooking time: 15 minutes

Servings: 4

Ingredients:

- 2 tablespoons olive oil 1 onion, diced
- 1 green bell pepper, diced
- 1 carrot, peeled and diced
- 4 garlic cloves, minced
- two 15-ounce cans black beans, drained and rinsed

- 2 cups vegetable stock
- ¼ teaspoon ground cumin
- 1 teaspoon sea salt
- ¼ cup chopped cilantro, for garnish

Directions:

1. In a large soup pot, heat the olive oil over medium-high heat until it shimmers.
2. Add the onion, bell pepper, and carrot and cook until the vegetables soften, about 5 minutes. Add garlic and cook until it is fragrant, about 30 seconds. Add the black beans, vegetable stock, cumin, and salt. Cook over medium-high heat, stirring occasionally, for about 10 minutes.
3. Remove from the heat. Using a potato masher, mash the beans lightly, leaving some chunks in the soup. For a smoother soup, process in a blender or food processor. Serve hot, garnished with cilantro.

Creamy Garlic-Spinach Rotini Soup

Preparation time: 10 minutes

Cooking time: 15 minutes

Servings: 4

Nutrition (2 cups)

- Calories: 207
- Protein: 11g
- Total fat: 5g
- Saturated fat: 1g
- Carbohydrates: 34g
- Fiber: 7g

Ingredients:

- 1 cup chopped mushrooms
- ¼ teaspoon plus a pinch salt
- 4 garlic cloves, minced, or 1 teaspoon garlic powder
- 2 peeled carrots or ½ red bell pepper, chopped

- 6 cups Economical Vegetable Broth or water
- Pinch freshly ground black pepper
- 1 cup rotini or gnocchi
- ¾ cup unsweetened nondairy milk
- ¼ cup nutritional yeast
- 2 cups chopped fresh spinach
- ¼ cup pitted black olives or sun-dried tomatoes, chopped
  Herbed Croutons, for topping (optional)
- 1 teaspoon olive oil

Directions:

1. Heat the olive oil in a large soup pot over medium-high heat.
2. Add the mushrooms and a pinch of salt. Sauté for about 4 minutes, until the mushrooms are softened. Add the garlic (if using freshand carrots, sauté for 1 minute more. Add the vegetable broth, remaining ¼ teaspoon of salt, and pepper (plus the garlic powder, if using). Bring to a boil and add the pasta. Cook for about 10 minutes, until the pasta is just cooked.
3. Turn off the heat and stir in the milk, nutritional yeast, spinach, and olives. Top with croutons (if using).
4. Leftovers will keep in an airtight container for up to 1 week in the refrigerator or up to 1 month in the freezer.

White and Wild Mushroom Barley Soup

Preparation time: 5 minutes

Cooking time: 50 minutes

Servings: 4 to 6

Ingredients:

- 1 tablespoon olive oil
- 1 medium onion, chopped
- 1 medium carrot, chopped
- 2 celery ribs, chopped
- 12 ounces white mushrooms, lightly rinsed, patted dry, and sliced
- 8 ounces cremini, shiitake, or other wild mushrooms, lightly rinsed, patted dry, and cut into 1/4-inch slices
- 1 cup pearl barley
- 7 cups vegetable or mushroom broth (homemade, store-bought, or water)
- 1 teaspoon dried dillweed

- Salt and freshly ground black pepper
- 2 tablespoons minced fresh parsley

Directions:

1. In a large soup pot, heat the oil over medium heat. Add the onion, carrot, and celery. Cover and cook until soft, about 10 minutes. Uncover and stir in the mushrooms, barley, broth, dillweed, and salt and pepper to taste. Bring to a boil, then reduce heat to low and simmer, uncovered, until the barley and vegetables are tender, about 40 minutes.
2. Add the parsley, taste, adjust seasonings if necessary, and serve.

Zucchini Vegan Bacon Lasagna

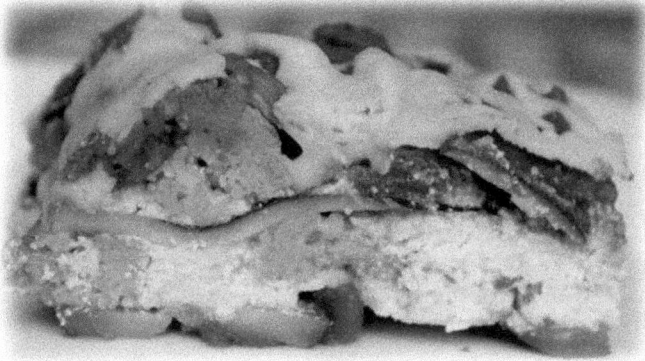

Preparation time: 15 minutes

Cooking time: 40 minutes

Serving: 4

Nutritional Values (Per Serving):

- Calories:417
- Total Fat: 36.4 g
- Saturated Fat: 15.9 g
- Total Carbs: 4 g

- Dietary Fiber:0 g
- Sugar: 1g
- Protein 20: g
- Sodium: 525 mg

Ingredients:

- 4 large yellow zucchinis
- Salt and black pepper to taste
- 1 tbsp lard
- ½ lb vegan bacon
- 1 tsp garlic powder 1 tsp onion powder
- 2 tbsp coconut flour
- ½ cup grated mozzarella cheese
- 1/3 cup cheddar cheese
- cups crumbled ricotta cheese
- 1 large egg
- cups unsweetened marinara sauce
- 1 tbsp Italian herb seasoning
- ¼ tsp red chili flakes
- ¼ cup fresh basil leaves

Directions:

1. Preheat the oven to 375 F and grease a 9 x 9-inch baking dish with cooking spray. Set aside.

2. Slice the zucchini into ¼ -inch strips, arrange on a flat surface and sprinkle generously with salt. Set aside to release liquid for 5 to 10 minutes. Pat dry with a paper towel and set aside.

3. Melt the lard in a large skillet over medium heat and add the vegan bacon. Cook until browned, 10 minutes. Set aside to cool.

4. In a medium bowl, evenly combine the garlic powder, onion powder, coconut flour, salt, black pepper, mozzarella cheese, half of the cheddar cheese, ricotta cheese, and egg. Set aside.

5. Add the Italian herb seasoning and red chili flakes to the marinara sauce and mix. Set aside.

6. Make a single layer of the zucchini in the baking dish; spread a quarter of the egg mixture on top, and a quarter of the marinara sauce. Repeat the layering process and sprinkle the top with the remaining cheddar cheese.

7. Bake in the oven for 30 minutes or until golden brown on top.

8. Remove the dish from the oven, allow cooling for 5 to 10 minutes, garnish with the basil leaves, slice and serve.

Black Bean Taco Salad Bowl

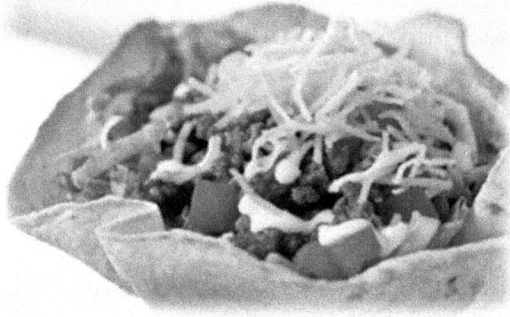

Preparation time: 15 minutes

Cooking time: 5 minutes

Servings: 3

Nutritional Values (Per Serving):

- Calories: 589
- Total fat: 14g
- Carbs: 101g
- Fiber: 20g
- Protein: 21g

Ingredients:

For the black bean salad

- 1 (14-ouncecan black beans, drained and rinsed, or 1½ cups cooked 1 cup corn kernels, fresh and blanched, or frozen and thawed
- ¼ cup fresh cilantro, or parsley, chopped
- Zest and juice of 1 lime
- 1 to 2 teaspoons chili powder
- Pinch sea salt
- 1½ cups cherry tomatoes, halved
- 1 red bell pepper, seeded and chopped
- 2 scallions, chopped

For 1 serving of tortilla chips

- 1 large whole-grain tortilla or wrap
- 1 teaspoon olive oil
- Pinch sea salt
- Pinch freshly ground black pepper
- Pinch dried oregano
- Pinch chili powder

For 1 bowl

- 1 cup fresh greens (lettuce, spinach, or whatever you like
- ¾ cup cooked quinoa, or brown rice, millet, or other whole grain

- ¼ cup chopped avocado, or Guacamole
- ¼ cup Fresh Mango Salsa

Directions:

For the black bean salad

1. Toss all the ingredients together in a large bowl.

Fort the tortilla chips

2. Brush the tortilla with olive oil, then sprinkle with salt, pepper, oregano, chili powder, and any other seasonings you like. Slice it into eighths like a pizza.
3. Transfer the tortilla pieces to a small baking sheet lined with parchment paper and put in the oven or toaster oven to toast or broil for 3 to 5 minutes, until browned. Keep an eye on them, as they can go from just barely done to burned very quickly.

For the bowl

4. Lay the greens in the bowl, top with the cooked quinoa, ⅓ of the black bean salad, the avocado, and salsa.

Romaine and Grape Tomato Salad with Avocado and Baby Peas

Preparation time: 15 minutes

Cooking time: 0 minutes

Servings: 4

Ingredients:

- 1 garlic clove, chopped
- 1 tablespoon chopped shallot
- 1/2 teaspoon dried basil
- 1/2 teaspoon salt
- 1/8 teaspoon freshly ground black pepper
- 1/4 teaspoon brown sugar (optional
- 3 tablespoons white wine vinegar
- 1/3 cup olive oil
- 1 medium head romaine lettuce, cut into 1/4-inch strips
- 12 ripe grape tomatoes, halved
- 1/2 cup frozen baby peas, thawed

- 8 kalamata olives, pitted
- 1 ripe Hass avocado

Directions:

1. In a blender or food processor, combine the garlic, shallot, basil, salt, pepper, sugar, and vinegar until smooth. Add the oil and blend until emulsified. Set aside.
2. In a large bowl, combine the lettuce, tomatoes, peas, and olives. Pit and peel the avocado and cut into 1/2-inch dice. Add to the bowl, along with enough dressing to lightly coat. Toss gently to combine and serve.

Warm Vegetable "Salad"

Preparation time: 10 minutes

Cooking time: 15 minutes

Servings: 4

Nutritional Values (Per Serving):

- Calories: 393
- Fat: 15g
- Protein: 10g
- Carbohydrates: 52g
- Fiber: 9g
- Sugar: 8g
- Sodium: 343mg

Ingredients:

- Salt for salting water, plus ½ teaspoon (optional)
- 4 red potatoes, quartered
- 1 pound carrots, sliced into ¼-inch-thick rounds
- 1 tablespoon extra-virgin olive oil (optional)
- 2 tablespoons lime juice

- 2 teaspoons dried dill
- ¼ teaspoon freshly ground black pepper
- 1 cup Cashew Cream or Parm-y Kale Pesto

Directions:

1. In a large pot, bring salted water to a boil. Add the potatoes and cook for 8 minutes. Add the carrots and continue to boil for another 8 minutes, until both the potatoes and carrots are crisp tender. Drain and return to the pot. Add the olive oil (if using), lime juice, dill, remaining ½ teaspoon of salt (if using), and pepper, and stir to coat well.

2. Divide the vegetables evenly among 4 single-compartment storage containers or wide-mouth pint glass jars, and spoon ¼ cup of cream or pesto over the vegetables in each. Let cool before sealing the lids.

Puttanesca Seitan and Spinach Salad

Preparation time: 5 minutes

Cooking time: 6 minutes

Servings: 4

Ingredients:

- 4 tablespoons olive oil
- 8 ounces seitan, homemade or store-bought, cut into 1⁄2-inch strips
- 3 garlic cloves, minced
- 1⁄2 cup kalamata olives, pitted and halved
- 1⁄2 cup green olives, pitted and halved
- 2 tablespoons capers
- 3 cups fresh baby spinach, cut into strips
- 11⁄2 cups ripe cherry tomatoes, halved
- 2 tablespoons balsamic vinegar
- 1⁄4 teaspoon salt (optional)
- 1⁄4 teaspoon freshly ground black pepper

- 2 tablespoons torn fresh basil leaves
- 2 tablespoons minced fresh parsley

Directions:

1. In a large skillet, heat 1 tablespoon of the oil over medium heat. Add the seitan and cook until browned on both sides, about 5 minutes. Add the garlic and cook until fragrant, about 30 seconds. Transfer to a large bowl and set aside to cool, about 15 minutes.

2. When the seitan has cooled to room temperature, add the kalamata and green olives, capers, spinach, and tomatoes. Set aside.

3. In a small bowl, combine the remaining 3 tablespoons oil with the vinegar, salt, and pepper. Whisk until blended, then pour the dressing over the salad. Add the basil and parsley, toss gently to combine, and serve.

Nori Snack Rolls

Preparation time: 5 minutes

Cooking time: 10 minutes

Servings: 4 rolls

Nutrition (1 roll):

- Calories: 79
- Total fat: 5g
- Carbs: 6g
- Fiber: 2g
- Protein: 4g

Ingredients:

- 2 tablespoons almond, cashew, peanut, or other nut butter
- 2 tablespoons tamari, or soy sauce
- 4 standard nori sheets
- 1 mushroom, sliced

- 1 tablespoon pickled ginger
- ½ cup grated carrots

Directions:

1. Preheat the oven to 350°F.
2. Mix together the nut butter and tamari until smooth and very thick. Lay out a nori sheet, rough side up, the long way.
3. Spread a thin line of the tamari mixture on the far end of the nori sheet, from side to side. Lay the mushroom slices, ginger, and carrots in a line at the other end (the end closest to you).
4. Fold the vegetables inside the nori, rolling toward the tahini mixture, which will seal the roll. Repeat to make 4 rolls.
5. Put on a baking sheet and bake for 8 to 10 minutes, or until the rolls are slightly browned and crispy at the ends. Let the rolls cool for a few minutes, then slice each roll into 3 smaller pieces.

Risotto Bites

Preparation time: 15 minutes

Cooking time: 20 minutes

Servings: 12 bites

Nutrition (6 bites):

- Calories: 100
- Fat: 2g
- Protein: 6g
- Carbohydrates: 17g
- Fiber: 5g
- Sugar: 2g
- Sodium: 165mg

Ingredients:

- ½ cup panko bread crumbs
- 1 teaspoon paprika
- 1 teaspoon chipotle powder or ground cayenne pepper 1½ cups cold Green Pea Risotto
- Nonstick cooking spray

Directions:

1. Preheat the oven to 425°F.
2. Line a baking sheet with parchment paper.
3. On a large plate, combine the panko, paprika, and chipotle powder. Set aside.
4. Roll 2 tablespoons of the risotto into a ball.
5. Gently roll in the bread crumbs, and place on the prepared baking sheet. Repeat to make a total of 12 balls.
6. Spritz the tops of the risotto bites with nonstick cooking spray and bake for 15 to 20 minutes, until they begin to brown. Cool completely before storing in a large airtight container in a single layer (add a piece of parchment paper for a second layeror in a plastic freezer bag.

Jicama and Guacamole

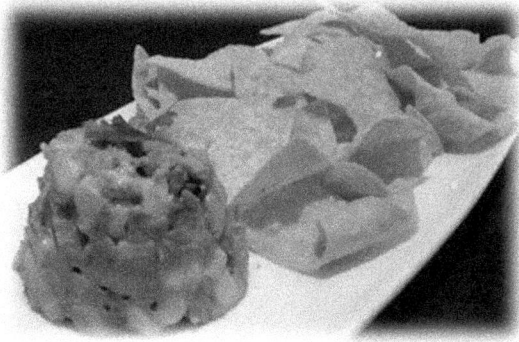

Preparation time: 15 minutes

Cooking time: 0 minutes

Servings: 4

Ingredients:

- juice of 1 lime, or 1 tablespoon prepared lime juice
- 2 hass avocados, peeled, pits removed, and cut into cubes
- ½ teaspoon sea salt
- ½ red onion, minced
- 1 garlic clove, minced
- ¼ cup chopped cilantro (optional)
- 1 jicama bulb, peeled and cut into matchsticks

Directions:

1. In a medium bowl, squeeze the lime juice over the top of the avocado and sprinkle with salt.
2. Lightly mash the avocado with a fork. Stir in the onion, garlic, and cilantro, if using.
3. Serve with slices of jicama to dip in guacamole.
4. To store, place plastic wrap over the bowl of guacamole and refrigerate. The guacamole will keep for about 2 days.

Curried Tofu "Egg Salad" Pitas

Preparation time: 15 minutes

Cooking time: 0 minutes

Servings: 4 sandwiches

Ingredients:

- 1 pound extra-firm tofu, drained and patted dry
- 1⁄2 cup vegan mayonnaise, homemade or store-bought
- 1⁄4 cup chopped mango chutney, homemade or store-bought
- 2 teaspoons Dijon mustard
- 1 tablespoon hot or mild curry powder
- 1 teaspoon salt
- 1⁄8 teaspoon ground cayenne
- ¾ cup shredded carrots
- 2 celery ribs, minced
- 1⁄4 cup minced red onion
- 8 small Boston or other soft lettuce leaves
- 4 7-inchwhole wheat pita breads, halved

Directions:

1. Crumble the tofu and place it in a large bowl. Add the mayonnaise, chutney, mustard, curry powder, salt, and cayenne, and stir well until thoroughly mixed.
2. Add the carrots, celery, and onion and stir to combine. Refrigerate for 30 minutes to allow the flavors to blend.
3. Tuck a lettuce leaf inside each pita pocket, spoon some tofu mixture on top of the lettuce, and serve.

Garden Patch Sandwiches On Multigrain Bread

Preparation time: 15 minutes

Cooking time: 0 minutes

Servings: 4 sandwiches

Ingredients:

- 1 pound extra-firm tofu, drained and patted dry
- 1 medium red bell pepper, finely chopped
- 1 celery rib, finely chopped
- 3 green onions, minced
- 1/4 cup shelled sunflower seeds
- 1/2 cup vegan mayonnaise, homemade or store-bought 1/2 teaspoon salt
- 1/2 teaspoon celery salt
- 1/4 teaspoon freshly ground black pepper
- 8 slices whole grain bread
- 4 (1/4-inchslices ripe tomato
- 4 lettuce leaves

Directions:

1. Crumble the tofu and place it in a large bowl. Add the bell pepper, celery, green onions, and sunflower seeds. Stir in the mayonnaise, salt, celery salt, and pepper and mix until well combined.

2. Toast the bread, if desired. Spread the mixture evenly onto 4 slices of the bread. Top each with a tomato slice, lettuce leaf, and the remaining bread. Cut the sandwiches diagonally in half and serve.

Maple-Walnut Oatmeal Cookies

Preparation time: 5 minutes

Cooking time: 10 minutes

Servings: about 2 dozen cookies

Ingredients:

- 1½ cups whole-grain flour
- 1 teaspoon baking powder
- ⅛ teaspoon salt
- 1 teaspoon ground cinnamon
- ¼ teaspoon ground nutmeg
- 1½ cups old-fashioned oats
- 1 cup chopped walnuts
- ½ cup vegan margarine, melted
- ½ cup pure maple syrup
- ¼ cup light brown sugar
- 2 teaspoons pure vanilla extract

Directions:

1. Preheat the oven to 375°F. In a large bowl, sift together the flour, baking powder, salt, cinnamon, and nutmeg. Stir in the oats and walnuts.

2. In a medium bowl, combine the margarine, maple syrup, sugar, and vanilla and mix well.

3. Add the wet ingredients to the dry ingredients: stirring to mix well.

4. Drop the cookie dough by the tablespoonful onto an ungreased baking sheet and press down slightly with a fork. Bake until browned, 10 to 12 minutes. Cool the cookies slightly before transferring to a wire rack to cool completely. Store in an airtight container.

Banana-Nut Bread Bars

Preparation time: 5 minutes

Cooking time: 30 minutes

Servings: 9 bars

Nutrition (1 bar):

- Calories: 73
- Fat: 1g
- Protein: 2g
- Carbohydrates: 15g
- Fiber: 2g
- Sugar: 5g
- Sodium: 129mg

Ingredients:

- Nonstick cooking spray (optional)
- 2 large ripe bananas
- 1 tablespoon maple syrup
- ½ teaspoon vanilla extract
- 2 cups old-fashioned rolled oats

- ½ teaspoons salt
- ¼ cup chopped walnuts

Directions:

1. Preheat the oven to 350°F. Lightly coat a 9-by-9-inch baking pan with nonstick cooking spray (if usingor line with parchment paper for oil-free baking.
2. In a medium bowl, mash the bananas with a fork. Add the maple syrup and vanilla extract and mix well. Add the oats, salt, and walnuts, mixing well.
3. Transfer the batter to the baking pan and bake for 25 to 30 minutes, until the top is crispy. Cool completely before slicing into 9 bars. Transfer to an airtight storage container or a large plastic bag.

Apple Crumble

Preparation time: 20 minutes

Cooking time: 25 minutes

Servings: 6

Nutrition:

- Calories: 356
- Total fat: 17g
- Carbs: 49g
- Fiber: 7g
- Protein: 7g

Ingredients:

For the filling

- 4 to 5 apples, cored and chopped (about 6 cups)
- ½ cup unsweetened applesauce, or ¼ cup water
- 2 to 3 tablespoons unrefined sugar (coconut, date, sucanat, maple syrup)
- 1 teaspoon ground cinnamon

- Pinch sea salt

For the crumble

- 2 tablespoons almond butter, or cashew or sunflower seed butter
- 2 tablespoons maple syrup
- 1½ cups rolled oats
- ½ cup walnuts, finely chopped
- ½ teaspoon ground cinnamon
- 2 to 3 tablespoons unrefined granular sugar (coconut, date, sucanat)

Directions:

1. Preheat the oven to 350°F. Put the apples and applesauce in an 8-inch-square baking dish, and sprinkle with the sugar, cinnamon, and salt. Toss to combine.
2. In a medium bowl, mix together the nut butter and maple syrup until smooth and creamy. Add the oats, walnuts, cinnamon, and sugar and stir to coat, using your hands if necessary. (If you have a small food processor, pulse the oats and walnuts together before adding them to the mix.
3. Sprinkle the topping over the apples, and put the dish in the oven.
4. Bake for 20 to 25 minutes, or until the fruit is soft and the topping is lightly browned.

Chocolate-Cranberry Oatmeal Cookies

Preparation time: 5 minutes

Cooking time: 15 minutes

Servings: about 2 dozen cookies

Ingredients:

- 1⁄2 cup vegan margarine
- 1 cup sugar
- 1⁄4 cup apple juice
- 1 cup whole-grain flour
- 1 teaspoon baking powder
- 1⁄2 teaspoon salt
- 1 teaspoon pure vanilla extract
- 1 cup old-fashioned oats
- 1⁄2 cup vegan semisweet chocolate chips
- 1⁄2 cup sweetened dried cranberries

Directions:

1. Preheat the oven to 375°F. In a large bowl, cream together the margarine and the sugar until light and fluffy. Blend in the juice.

2. Add the flour, baking powder, salt, and vanilla, blending well. Stir in the oats, chocolate chips, and cranberries and mix well.

3. Drop the dough from a teaspoon onto an ungreased baking sheet. Bake until nicely browned, about 15 minutes. Cool the cookies slightly before transferring to a wire rack to cool completely. Store in an airtight container.

Cashew-Chocolate Truffles

Preparation time: 15 minutes

Cooking time: 0 minutes • plus 1 hour to set

Servings: 12 truffles

Nutrition (1 truffle):

- Calories 238
- Fat: 18g
- Protein: 3g
- Carbohydrates: 16g
- Fiber: 4g
- Sugar: 9g
- Sodium: 9mg

Ingredients:

- 1 cup raw cashews, soaked in water overnight
- ¾ cup pitted dates
- 2 tablespoons coconut oil
- 1 cup unsweetened shredded coconut, divided
- 1 to 2 tablespoons cocoa powder, to taste

Directions:

1. In a food processor, combine the cashews, dates, coconut oil, ½ cup of shredded coconut, and cocoa powder. Pulse until fully incorporated; it will resemble chunky cookie dough. Spread the remaining ½ cup of shredded coconut on a plate.

2. Form the mixture into tablespoon-size balls and roll on the plate to cover with the shredded coconut. Transfer to a parchment paper–lined plate or baking sheet. Repeat to make 12 truffles.

3. Place the truffles in the refrigerator for 1 hour to set. Transfer the truffles to a storage container or freezer-safe bag and seal.

Banana Chocolate Cupcakes

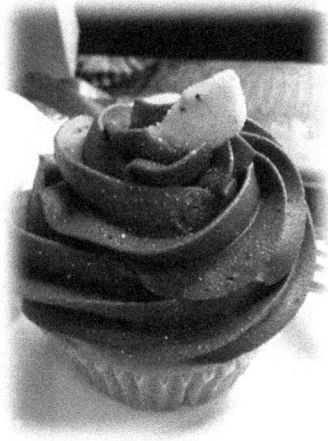

Preparation time: 20 minutes

Cooking time: 20 minutes

Servings: 12 cupcakes

Nutrition (1 cupcake):

- Calories: 215
- Total fat: 6g
- Carbs: 39g
- Fiber: 9g
- Protein: 6g

Ingredients:

- 3 medium bananas
- 1 cup non-dairy milk
- 2 tablespoons almond butter
- 1 teaspoon apple cider vinegar
- 1 teaspoon pure vanilla extract
- 1¼ cups whole-wheat flour
- ½ cup rolled oats
- ¼ cup coconut sugar (optional)
- 1 teaspoon baking powder
- ½ teaspoon baking soda
- ½ cup unsweetened cocoa powder
- ¼ cup chia seeds, or sesame seeds
- Pinch sea salt
- ¼ cup dark chocolate chips, dried cranberries, or raisins (optional)

Directions:

1. Preheat the oven to 350°F. Lightly grease the cups of two 6-cup muffin tins or line with paper muffin cups.
2. Put the bananas, milk, almond butter, vinegar, and vanilla in a blender and purée until smooth. Or stir together in a large bowl until smooth and creamy.

3. Put the flour, oats, sugar (if using), baking powder, baking soda, cocoa powder, chia seeds, salt, and chocolate chips in another large bowl, and stir to combine. Mix together the wet and dry ingredients, stirring as little as possible. Spoon into muffin cups, and bake for 20 to 25 minutes. Take the cupcakes out of the oven and let them cool fully before taking out of the muffin tins, since they'll be very moist.

Minty Fruit Salad

Preparation time: 15 minutes

Cooking time: 5 minutes

Servings: 4

Nutritional Values (Per Serving):

- Calories: 138
- Fat: 1g
- Protein: 2g
- Carbohydrates: 34g
- Fiber: 8g
- Sugar: 22g
- Sodium: 6mg

Ingredients:

- ¼ cup lemon juice (about 2 small lemons)
- 4 teaspoons maple syrup or agave syrup
- 2 cups chopped pineapple
- 2 cups chopped strawberries
- 2 cups raspberries

- 1 cup blueberries
- 8 fresh mint leaves

Directions:

1. Beginning with 1 mason jar, add the ingredients in this order: 1 tablespoon of lemon juice, 1 teaspoon of maple syrup, ½ cup of pineapple, ½ cup of strawberries, ½ cup of raspberries, ¼ cup of blueberries, and 2 mint leaves.
2. Repeat to fill 3 more jars. Close the jars tightly with lids.
3. Place the airtight jars in the refrigerator for up to 3 days.

Sesame Cookies

Preparation time: 15 minutes

Cooking time: 0 minutes

Servings: 3 dozen cookies

Ingredients:

- ¾ cup vegan margarine, softened
- ½ cup light brown sugar
- 1 teaspoon pure vanilla extract
- 2 tablespoons pure maple syrup
- ¼ teaspoon salt
- 2 cups whole-grain flour
- ¾ cup sesame seeds, lightly toasted

Directions:

1. In a large bowl, cream together the margarine and sugar until light and fluffy. Blend in the vanilla, maple syrup, and salt. Stir in the flour and sesame seeds and mix well.

2. Roll the dough into a cylinder about 2 inches in diameter. Wrap it in plastic wrap and refrigerate for 1 hour or longer. Preheat the oven to 325°F.

3. Slice the cookie dough into 1/8-inch-thick rounds and arrange on an ungreased baking sheet about 2 inches apart. Bake until light brown, about 12 minutes. When completely cool, store in an airtight container.

Mango Coconut Cream Pie

Preparation time: 20 minutes • chill time: 30 minutes

Servings: 8

Nutrition (1 slice):

- Calories: 427
- Total fat: 28g
- Carbs: 45g
- Fiber: 6g
- Protein: 8g

Ingredients:

For the crust

- ½ cup rolled oats 1 cup cashews
- 1 cup soft pitted dates

For the filling

- 1cup canned coconut milk
- ½ cup water

- 2large mangos, peeled and chopped, or about 2 cups frozen chunks
- ½ cup unsweetened shredded coconut

Directions:

1. Put all the crust ingredients in a food processor and pulse until it holds together. If you don't have a food processor, chop everything as finely as possible and use ½ cup cashew or almond butter in place of half the cashews. Press the mixture down firmly into an 8-inch pie or springform pan.
2. Put the all filling ingredients:in a blender and purée until smooth (about 1 minute). It should be very thick, so you may have to stop and stir until it's smooth.
3. Pour the filling into the crust, use a rubber spatula to smooth the top, and put the pie in the freezer until set, about 30 minutes. Once frozen, it should be set out for about 15 minutes to soften before serving.
4. Top with a batch of Coconut Whipped Cream scooped on top of the pie once it's set. Finish it off with a sprinkling of toasted shredded coconut.

Avocado Pesto Zoodles

Preparation time: 10 minutes

Cooking time: 10 minutes

Servings: 2

Nutritional Values (Per Serving):

- Calories 404
- Fat, 31g
- Protein 14g
- Carbs 27g
- Fiber 14g
- Sugar 7g
- Sodium 766mg

Ingredients:

- 1 avocado, halved
- 1 tablespoon pine nuts

- ½ cup fresh basil
- 2 teaspoons olive oil
- 4 medium zucchini, spiralized
- 1 tablespoon minced garlic
- 4 tablespoons shredded Parmesan cheese
- ½ teaspoon salt
- ½ teaspoon freshly ground black pepper

Directions:

1. In the bowl of a food processor, combine the avocados, pine nuts, and basil. Pulse until a paste forms, using a few tablespoons of water to thin the consistency if necessary.
2. Heat a medium skillet over medium-high heat and pour in the olive oil. Add the zoodles and garlic and sauté for 5 to 7 minutes.
3. Add the avocado pesto to the skillet and stir until well combined.
4. Cook for an additional 1 to 2 minutes and top with the Parmesan cheese, salt, and pepper.

Cauliflower Rice

Preparation time: 15 minutes

Cooking time: 10 minutes

Servings: 2

Nutritional Values (Per Serving):

- Calories 74
- Fat 6g
- Protein 1g
- Carbs 4g
- Fiber 2g
- Sugar 2g
- Sodium 642mg

Ingredients:

- ½ head cauliflower
- 1 tablespoon grass-fed butter
- ½ teaspoon salt
- ⅛ teaspoon freshly ground black pepper

Directions:

1. Wash the cauliflower under cold water. Pat dry with paper towels.
2. Chop the cauliflower into 1-inch pieces and put in a food processor. Pulse until the size of small rice.
3. Place a small griddle over medium-high heat. Melt the butter and add the cauliflower. Season with the salt and pepper and cook for 7 to 8 minutes, or until the cauliflower is tender.

Avocado Lime Dressing

Preparation time: 5 minutes

Cooking time: 0 minutes

Servings: 6

Nutritions:

- Calories 146
- Fat 14g
- Protein 1g
- Carbs 4g
- Fiber 2g
- Sugar 0g
- Sodium 51mg

Ingredients:

- 1 avocado, halved
- Leaves of 1 bunch fresh cilantro
- ¼ cup avocado oil
- 2 tablespoons water
- 2 tablespoons freshly squeezed lime juice

- 1 garlic clove, peeled
- 1 teaspoon garlic salt

Directions:

1. Combine all the ingredients in a high-powered blender or a food processor and pulse until thoroughly combined, 2 to 3 minutes. Transfer to a small mason jar and store in the refrigerator until ready to use.

Quick and Easy Ranch Dip

Preparation time: 10 minutes plus 4hrs chill time

Cooking time: 0 minutes

Servings: 12

Nutritions:

- Calories 79
- Fat 7g
- Protein 2g
- Carbs: 2g
- Fiber 0g
- Sugar 2g
- Sodium 109mg

Ingredients:

- 1 cup heavy (whipping) cream
- 1 tablespoon white distilled vinegar
- ¾ cup plain full-fat Greek yogurt
- 1 teaspoon freshly squeezed lemon juice
- 2 teaspoons dried parsley

- 1 teaspoon dried dill
- 1 teaspoon dried chives
- ½ teaspoon garlic powder
- ½ teaspoon onion powder
- ½ teaspoon salt
- ¼ teaspoon freshly ground black pepper

Directions:

1. In a quart-size canning jar, combine the heavy cream and vinegar. Set aside for 5 minutes.
2. Add the Greek yogurt and lemon juice and stir (or shake the jar) well.
3. Add the parsley, dill, chives, garlic powder, onion powder, salt, and pepper, and stir until thoroughly mixed.
4. Put the lid on the jar and place in the refrigerator for 4 hours or overnight for the flavors to combine.

Easy Keto Bread

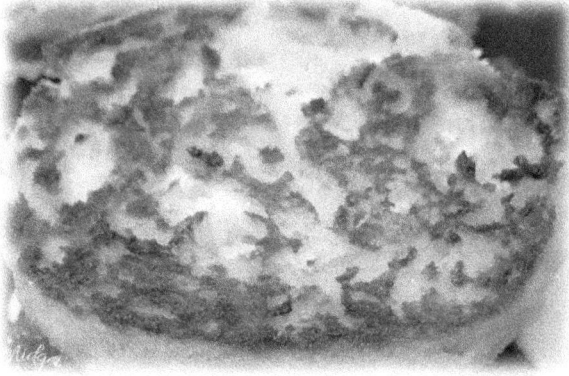

Preparation time: 15 minutes

Cooking time: 1 hour & 15 minutes

Servings: 4

Nutritions:

- Calories 121
- Fat 9g
- Protein 5g
- Carbs 5g
- Fiber 3g
- Sugar 0g
- Sodium 86mg

Ingredients:

- Nonstick cooking spray
- 1 cup blanched almond flour
- ¼ cup coconut flour
- 2 teaspoons baking powder
- ¼ teaspoon salt
- ⅓ cup coconut oil, melted
- 12 egg whites

Directions:

1. Preheat the oven to 350°F. Spray a loaf pan with cooking spray, making sure to cover the interior corners and sides completely.
2. In the bowl of a food processor, combine the almond flour, coconut flour, baking powder, and salt. Pulse until well combined.
3. Add the coconut oil and pulse again until a crumble forms. Set aside.
4. In a large bowl, use a handheld electric mixer to beat the egg whites until stiff peaks form, about 10 minutes. (You can add ¼ teaspoon of cream of tartar to help the egg whites whip up faster.)
5. Add half the whipped egg whites to the food processor. Pulse a few times. Don't overbeat or you will deflate the egg whites.

6. Bit by bit, add the flour mixture to the remaining egg whites in the large bowl. Fold the flour into the egg whites very gently until well combined.
7. Spread the batter in the prepared bread pan.
8. Bake for 40 minutes, or until the top of the bread is lightly browned.
9. Place a layer of aluminum foil over the top of the bread (to avoid overbrowning) and cook for an additional 35 minutes.
10. Transfer the bread to a wire rack. When cooled, slice evenly.

www.ingramcontent.com/pod-product-compliance
Lightning Source LLC
Chambersburg PA
CBHW050748030426
42336CB00012B/1717